HENDA'S LAW

Henda's Law: Dense Breast Tissue—What You Need to Know

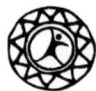

Copyright © 2018 Jabulani House
www.HendasLaw.com

JABULANI
HOUSE

FLUENCY
TELLING STORIES THAT MATTER

Produced with the assistance of Fluency Organization, Inc.
Graphic design: Inkwell Creative
Cover: André Provedel
Photographer: Greg Blomberg

Printed in the United States of America

To everyone whose life has been affected by breast cancer.

Also available on Amazon by Henda Salmeron:
Grit Under My Nails: A Memoir in Three Acts

A portion of the net proceeds from the sale of this book
will be donated to The Henda Salmeron Foundation.

SUPPORT FOR HENDA'S LAW

"As a practicing oncologist focusing on breast cancer, I see many patients with dense breasts. Until recently, the patients with dense breasts were not adequately evaluated. With gratitude to Henda Salmeron for establishing Henda's Law, we are now truly encompassing the meaning of "early detection." Many women are not aware of the meaning of dense breasts. This is not a physical diagnosis; it is a radiographical diagnosis only seen on mammograms. It is crucial that we additionally evaluate dense breasts with ultrasounds or MRI in order to detect occult disease. Empowering women with the knowledge that they have dense breasts and that they need further evaluation is due to Henda's pioneering work and tireless fight. By changing the law, we are making a better tomorrow for all women with dense breasts. We are grateful to Henda and her work in saving women's lives—she is not only a survivor but also a true example of a thriver."

—**S. J. Vukelja, M.D., F.A.C.P.,** Texas Oncology, Tyler, Texas, Medical Oncologist, Practice limited to Hematology and Medical Oncology

"Henda's Law has provided health care professionals like myself with both the means and justification necessary to more effectively promote women's awareness of their breast density, thereby empowering women to seek more effective screening strategies to detect breast cancer at its earliest and most treatable stage."

—**John Larrinaga, M.D.,** Medical Director, Ross Breast Center, Christus Trinity Mother Frances Health System

"Prior to Henda's Law, breast density was largely ignored by the radiology community, despite the fact that 1/4 to 1/3 of small breast cancers remained mammographically hidden by dense breast tissue. Since the advent of the law, however, this topic as received national attention and led to the passage of similar laws in states from coast-to-coast. Henda has prodded the medical community nation-wide to consider how they treat patients when it comes to early detection of breast cancer and yearly mammograms."

—**Michael J. Ulissey MD, FACR,**
Board of Directors: Texas Radiological Society,
Adjunct Professor of Radiology: The University of Texas Health Sciences Center

"Dr. Roshni Rao, assistant professor of surgery at the University of Texas Southwestern Medical Center in Dallas, said one woman's personal battle with breast cancer was the inspiration for Henda's Law—a Texas law named for Henda Salmeron that requires women to be informed about their breast tissue's density and the limitations of mammography in certain cases."

—**UPI,** United Press International Health News

HENDA SALMERON

HENDA'S LAW

DENSE BREAST TISSUE
What You NEED To Know!

TABLE OF CONTENTS

ABOUT THE AUTHOR

Henda's Law changed the standard of care for every woman in the State of Texas on June 17, 2011 when Governor Perry signed the bill. House Bill 2102, by State law, requires every mammography provider to specifically notify women that they have dense breast tissue and the increased risks associated therewith. The law is named after Henda Salmeron, the "Maverick Mom, Survivor, Author, Investor, and Award-Winning Real Estate Broker," who created, lobbied, and passed Texas HB-2102. Since its ratification in the State of Texas in 2011 it has directly influenced the subsequent passing and/or introduction of sister bills across the United States. The law is responsible for alerting millions of women about their breast density and their increased potential for undetected breast tumors in dense breasts. Furthermore, it has educated them about the limitations of mammography as it relates to dense breasts and the importance of consulting with their physicians about the benefit of supplemental screening based on their individual risk factors.

This book details the events leading to Henda's surprising cancer diagnosis, treatment, and how she became a pioneer and accidental lobbyist for one of the most important breast cancer bills ever passed in the United States of America. The content is excerpted from her memoir: *Grit Under My Nails: A Memoir in Three Acts.*

A breast cancer survivor and activist since 2009, Henda is an award-winning real estate broker with Dave Perry-Miller Real Estate in Dallas, Texas. She arrived in the United States in 1990 with only a few possessions and the American dream of achieving success. She has served on the Susan G. Komen Dallas County board and is a current advisory board member of The Bridge Breast Network. A lifetime member of Leadership Dallas, Henda contributes her time and effort to many other causes locally and nationally.

As an avid adventurist, certified diver, ultra-extreme endurance athlete, and adrenaline driven type A, Henda regularly travels the globe, creating a lifetime of memories both under and above the water. She has never met a challenge she hasn't loved and seeks fun and happiness every day. In addition to her favorite job—being her kids' mom—she has added author and inspirational speaker to her resumé.

Henda was honored by the State of Texas and the House of Representatives in 2010 for her information campaign regarding dense breast tissue. She also received special recognition from the City of Dallas for her community efforts.

Visit www.HendasLaw.com for more information regarding dense breast tissue.

CALL TO ACTION
Henda's Law Re-Awareness Campaign

HendasLaw.com leverages the influence of Henda's Law to bring continued awareness to dense breast tissue and its impact on breast cancer. The battle is not over, and breast cancer still affects many women across the country. Henda's Law is calling all mothers, daughters, and the men who love them to continue the fight by registering your support at www.HendasLaw.com.

Henda's Law Ongoing Mission:

- Educate women about the importance of knowing their breast density
- Encourage annual screening for women after forty—3D mammography is now the standard of care in Texas
- Collect electronic signatures for support. Together we can drive change at a federal level for consistent density disclosure for ALL states and the women in the Armed Forces
  - FDA must modify the Mammography Quality Standards Act to account for screening dense breast tissue
  - US Senators and members of Congress must support and pass the Breast Density and Mammography Reporting Act of 2017—House Bill H.R. 4122 and Senate Bill S.2006

Get Involved Right Now!

Register at www.HendasLaw.com
or text "FAN HENDA" to 609-375-0446

The Messenger

WHAT IS ON YOUR bucket list? You know. Those things we want to do before our time is up. Mine is much longer than my daily to-do list. I fancy winning the lottery so I can tick each one of them off: Summit Kilimanjaro. Trek the Australian Outback. Set foot on Antarctica. Dance the salsa in Cali, Colombia. Watch the polar bears in Churchill, Manitoba. Scuba Kona and Hawaii's famed Manta Ray night dive. Hike across Iceland. Take the train from Moscow to Vladivostok. Ride with the great wildebeest migration from the Serengeti to the Maasai Mara—on horseback! Munch on street food in Marrakesh, Morocco. Scuba dive the annual sardine run in Durban, South Africa. Billions of sardines move northward from the cold Agulhas Bank near Cape Town toward Mozambique. During this ocean spectacle thousands of dolphins chase the sardines and drive them into tight circles. It becomes the frenzied feeding ground of predators including sharks, whales, game fish, birds, and seals. I want to see it! Sigh. This is just the tip of my list for exploring and experiencing earth's bounty before my hourglass is empty.

In early May 2009 I was fortunate to dive in Placencia, Belize. It was during the annual spring migration of the whale sharks— another dive I wanted to check off. I was warned about it being challenging because some divers sense extreme disorientation. The dive occurs in bottomless blue open water in the absence of reefs, walls, or the ocean floor for guidance. I was uncertain how I would react and shared my unease with the dive master just before splashing overboard. He stayed close by, holding eye contact as we descended.

As suspected, I had an immediate claustrophobic feeling because I lost my reference point and felt as if I was drowning in cobalt. Freaked out, I briefly contemplated aborting the dive when the dive master left my side to assist another panicked diver in the group.

I coerced myself to just breathe as I slowly relaxed and surrendered to the richest sapphire I had ever seen. The concentrated blue was dotted with millions of white specks of plankton that gave me the feeling of floating among the stars in space. Our descent continued to approximately 100 feet. The ocean extended more than 3,300 feet beneath us where thousands upon thousands of

17

Cubera snapper spawned. The whale sharks came to Placencia during the spring to feast on these snapper spawn as well as other small fish and plankton. The gentle giants were filter feeders and totally docile beasts. Almost the size of school buses, they were also intimidating. Like all things untamed, we were warned there was no guarantee that we would spot any during our estimated 45-minute dive.

From the depths beneath me, an enormous shadow suddenly appeared. "Whale shark!" I futilely shouted aloud through my regulator as the animal came closer. Prior to the dive we were also cautioned about stiff fines if we tried to approach or touch a whale shark. But nobody had explained what to do when a whale shark approached you! Mistaking my fellow divers' air bubbles for spawn, the whale shark tried eating the bubbles from our regulators in a curious and playful way. He weaved through the divers and even nipped at some of their tanks. I took photographs as fast as I could and feverishly hoped that at least one might capture this immense creature.

Suddenly the whale shark turned right toward me! I hung motionless in the water. Luckily my camera was attached to my BC jacket as I dropped it by my side. In seconds he was mere inches away from my face. Staring into his eyes, my thoughts were suspended in the timeless space surrounding us. I slowly raised my hands and lightly ran them over his mouth that was big enough to swallow me. I then gently pushed him to one side, and he glided effortlessly underneath me. As I watched him disappear into the abyss, I had to blink very hard to stop tears from running down my cheeks and fogging my dive mask.

The dive occurred exactly thirty days before I felt a little lump in my right breast in late May. During the next year there would be many times when I would transport myself back to this moment when the whale shark and I locked eyes. I would come to think of him as a messenger sent to give me the courage I would require to run the course. It felt as if I had looked into the eyes of God.

Adventurous
Crazy
Beautiful

Wishes to go where people don't just say Merry Christmas
Dreams of changing the world
Wants to explore
Who loves to travel

Who fears cockroaches
Who is afraid of heights
Who likes to run
Who believes in a difference

Who loves Rooibos tea
Who loves to scuba dive
Who loves nature and the outdoors
Who loves South Africa

Who plans to stay successful in life
Who plans to be different
Who loves to laugh
Whose final destination is heaven

My mom, Henda

— DOMINIQUE SALMERON'S FIFTH-
GRADE MOTHER'S DAY POEM, 2012

East Texas in Springtime

T HE GUINEA FOWLS PLAYED chase through the vineyard.
Their dark grey feathers glistened in the sun, and the dense

white spots covering their plumage reminded me of the speckled coat of a whale shark. The female's two-syllable call "come-back, come- back" transported me to the farm in Makwassie in South Africa. As I watched them scurry around the vines looking for insects, I appreciated what a delightful way it was to enjoy my Sunday morning at a winery in East Texas.

The breeze gently lifted the young green grapevines, and I could sense the earth's anticipation of the fruit forming within. Row upon row the vines were cuffed to their trellises, training their tender growth to obey how the vintner wanted them to spread. Restricted but free simultaneously, it was a great study of the dichotomy I found within. With a craving to be wild and free, I was also bound to my reality. Cursed with the acute longing to explore the earth far and wide, the day-to-day requirements of existing seemed so restrictive.

I was in Tyler, Texas, to speak at a 2015 breast cancer conference. My layman's topic amid oncologists, radiologists, and breast surgeons? How pink became my badge of hope and courage. Combining the passion of red with the purity of white, pink comes in many shades. My wardrobe today holds an extensive assortment of the many tones of pink, from the lightest blush to a blazing hot pink coat daring a cold winter's day away. As I reflected on how I had come to this point, I was brought back six years earlier to a June morning in 2009.

June 7, 8:35 a.m.: "Henda, I'm so sorry but the biopsy confirmed you have breast cancer. So far the pathology shows it's the most treatable type. It looks like the tumor is small, and we caught it early."

In an instant my forty-two-year-old life was disrupted. While living my Dallas routine I had been oblivious to the time bomb slowly ticking against my breastbone. Pink ribbons and breast cancer happened to other people and older women, and until then it was not part of my reality. I had annual mammograms. In fact, just a few months earlier in December 2008, I'd had my fourth clear one. Like many women, I considered a mammogram foolproof. Although I knew that one in eight women will get the news none of us wants to hear, I had never considered drawing the "C" card.

What would have happened to me had I not decided in early spring 2009 to alter my "over" and "un" course—overweight and overstressed, unfit and unhealthy? After years of working fifteen-hour days it was time to suspend my slide into a few extra pounds and elevated blood pressure. Going to the gym held no appeal, nor did running or any of the usual boring conditioning options. My house was near the shores of White Rock Lake in Dallas and rowing turned out to be the key to unlocking a healthier me. While watching the sculls slice the water against the setting sun, I was inspired to learn how to sit on a twelve-inch banana peel with two oars and repeat the same feat. My friend Sam introduced me to Darvin, a local fitness guy. Between the two they worked out a health regime that included rowing on the water and on the indoor rowers. Within eight weeks twelve pounds melted away and a leaner me emerged. And a surprise bonus! A tiny lump, as hard as a pea, I found in my right breast.

When I voiced my concerns about what I had felt in my breast, my doctor reminded me that I'd just had a clear mammogram a few months earlier. Fortune placed me next to my mother-in-law, who was also a Ph.D. nurse, at a family dinner two weeks later. I confided in her about my lumpy friend and what the doctor had said. Both her message and her voice are as clear today as they were then.

May 23, 8:05 p.m.: "Henda, no lump is nothing. Have it checked again!"

Per her advice, I called my doctor soon afterward and begged her to please check the lump even though it might be benign. She ordered another mammogram, which was clear again. The screening clinic then wanted to send me home. By now the little voice in my head had become a loud and insistent cry. I refused to leave without checking further. A subsequent sonogram revealed a shadow of enough concern to warrant a needle biopsy. Looking back, I knew I had cancer when I felt the unyielding mass that didn't belong in my breast.

I was diagnosed with breast cancer on June 7 and transferred the next day to the University of Texas Southwestern Medical Center in Dallas. Considered one of the very top hospitals with a National Cancer Institute designation, they performed another mammogram, sonogram, and MRI. In the waiting room I had my first brush with pink, soon to become my favorite color. I was the young one in a room filled with grandmothers. In our bubblegum pink hospital frocks, we resembled an army dressed in really bad uniforms.

The MRI indicated that the cancer had spread to my lymph nodes. The radiologist performing the lymph node biopsy was a kind person who was not about to lie to me. He offered me the one-in-a-million consolation prize: if the MRI was incorrect, and my lymph nodes were not involved, my case would be included in the radiology literature of the medical school. No joke. Tell me again how I drew this card?

While I waited for the sonogram, tears ran down my cheeks unchecked. I almost sobbed without restraint when the nurse offered me her own stash of tissues while gently pointing out how hers were softer than the hospital-issued brand. The unreal sequence of events over the past twenty-four hours had dealt me a blow that left me in a zombie trance.

I adore roller coasters. Especially the kind when your throat gets hoarse from your blood-chilling screams as you plunge down the steepest hills into the tightest curves. There are few other places where your own screams are part of such fun. This self-induced punishment always leaves me with less emotional baggage than when I arrived. I wanted to scream that day in the waiting room at the top of my lungs because I was petrified and had no idea of the many twists and turns ahead. More than anything I wanted to get the hell out of the line and not go on the ride. Ever. However, destiny had other plans in store.

June 9, 2:05 p.m.: "Mrs. Salmeron, this is Dr. Rao with UT Southwestern. Is this a good time, and are you sitting down?"

Seriously. Can we please agree that no conversation should start that way? It was the moment that changed everything forever. Dr. Rao, my oncologist surgeon, broke the news to me gently. My tumor was not small, and my cancer was not in an early stage. She wanted me to come back to the hospital right away. We had to consider possibly starting chemo to shrink the four-centimeter tumor before she felt comfortable removing it.

June 9, 3:00 p.m.: Driving back to the hospital. You have to be kidding me! This is not happening! I have two little kids. Would I see them graduate from elementary school? How do I tell them that their mother could be dying? Am I going to die? How did this happen? How did a mammogram miss a tumor the diameter of a golf ball?

I despise cockroaches. Unequivocally, I hate them. They terrify me. The boarding house I lived in with my mother when I was a little girl was roach infested, and they crawled everywhere. Their antennae were always searching for my skin in the dark. Later as a student in boarding school, we had a perpetual roach problem in the bathrooms. You would not dare to walk barefoot in the middle of the night out of terror of stepping on one. I always imagined the "crunch-crunch" if you squashed the little bastards under your shoes. Ugh! I know Pixar tried to make them lovable. To me they are, and always will be, the creepy, scary monster insects from my childhood. My kids can vouch that I run screaming for the nearest chair to climb whenever I see one in my house today.

Apart from cockroaches, darkness had also scared me for decades. Not just any kind of night. The nights when I had to turn the lights out and go to bed by myself. I felt defenseless, certain that some deranged person would attack me while I was asleep. Remember my scissors- clutching nights? Certainly there should be no surprise about this phobia! Additionally, it didn't help that since fourth grade, I'd slept in dormitories surrounded by other warm bodies and in touching distance of another person.

My cancer diagnosis ushered in another awareness of fear— the dread of exhaling my last breath. This was a different league altogether. Suddenly the clichés of living and dying became personally relevant. Like a slo-mo flashback to Nicky's death, my own mortality was staring me down. For one who once dreaded the dark, driving back to the hospital on June 9, 2009, was one of my darkest days.

June 9, 4:05 p.m.: DENSE BREAST TISSUE . . . Huh? WTF!

I had never heard those three words strung together. Seriously? Bet you have never heard them either. Try saying "dense breast tissue" a few times fast. It reminds me of a tongue twister like "Sally sells seashells by the seashore." Wish I'd met the person that coined the phrase. Could they have come up instead with "solid," "impenetrable," or "thick" as synonyms to describe breast tissue?

I learned at the hospital that I had very dense breasts and that it was "not the standard of care" to inform women about their breast density. Oh, and by the way, a mammogram can miss a tumor in dense breasts 40% of the time. And, oh yeah, sorry to seem still bewildered, but more than half of women have dense breasts. Those are not small numbers! I'm not making this stuff up. Seriously. Until that moment I had thought "dense" meant "stupid."

It was like a very poorly scripted B-movie, bad jokes and all. I had a baseline mammogram at age thirty-five and faithfully had a mammogram every year beginning at age forty. All my mammograms clearly indicated that I had dense breast tissue, which is why it was inconceivable to me that no one had ever told me.

Are you ready for Breast Tissue 101? There is a quiz at the end of the book so you ought to pay close attention for the next few paragraphs. I still feel like sticking my fingers in my ears and going "la- la-la-la-la," so I know how you are going to feel in about two minutes! Only a mammogram can reveal the density of a woman's breast tissue. It has nothing to do with your breast size or how your breasts feel. Breast density refers to the proportion of fat and tissue in your breasts. Dense breasts have less fat, and low-density breasts have less tissue and more fat. Still with me? And this fat is not like your tummy or thigh fat that you can lose with a diet. You cannot change your combination of fat and tissue by lifting weights either.

One of the limitations of a mammogram is that dense breast tissue appears as a tight white web on a mammogram, while the tumors that mammography tries to detect are also white. How do you find a tumor on a mammogram when your breasts are dense? Try spotting a snowball in a blizzard. Or find a polar bear in the snow. It is white on white and impossible to see!

Don't get me wrong. Mammograms save lives. Until we can pee on a stick one day for cancer screening, they are the most cost-effective tools in our arsenal on the war against breast cancer. But they are not foolproof. Women must get screened regularly and know their breasts. As advocates of their own health, based on individual risk factors and discussions with their physicians, women should decide what else is prudent.

Don't I sound like a breast density pamphlet or infomercial? The number one reason women don't get screened is fright. Most women are afraid to get the results. Hell. I so totally get it. By the time I left the hospital on the day of my diagnosis, I was a brand-new expert about a subject I'd have rather stayed oblivious about.

June 10, 6:50 a.m.: Screw cancer.

I didn't bother going to bed the night before and had never felt so adrift, isolated, and frightened. I'd received a possible death sentence, and although adversity had been a close friend since I was young, I had no idea what to do. From one hour to the next, it was like an alien invasion of worry that wasn't there before. Terrible "what if" scenarios popped up in little crop circles in my head overnight. Apart from my own demise, I dreaded leaving my two little kids without their mother. Oh, my God. They were only eight and ten. How could this be happening? Hours into this purgatory, some clarity slowly surfaced. I. Am. Not. A. Quitter. And. I. Am. Not. Dead. Yet.

When daylight trickled across my backyard, I silently swore that I would not rest until I changed the "standard of care." All women deserved an equal opportunity to an early breast cancer diagnosis. By not telling us about our breast density, we lose that chance and could possibly lose our lives! I vowed that was *not* good enough.

Unbeknown to me, in the days, weeks, and months following this night of utter hell, fighting for this cause would become my saving grace. Like a drowning man I grabbed on to it. I redirected and funneled all the anger, frustration, and terror of my diagnosis into this one focal point. This budding crusade against cancer and the establishment created the illusion that I was in control. Those hours from midnight to dawn split me apart and fundamental change from this tender place was launched. Only years later would I fully understand its scope.

June 10, 10:00 a.m.: Mr. Vaught, my name is Henda Salmeron. I had to look you up online, as I didn't know who my local state representative was. And I'm sorry, but I also didn't vote for you. Mr. Vaught, I need you to, no . . . actually . . . I beg you . . . please help me change the standard of care for women with dense breast tissue!

I told Texas Representative Allen Vaught my story and pointed out some of what I'd already learned, namely that almost half of premenopausal women have dense breast tissue. I reminded him we were mothers, sisters, cousins, friends, wives, and often younger women who deserved to know the truth about our breasts. We were not a small minority! He agreed to consider the case. Unclear about the future, I felt that I'd at least tossed my first pebble.

June 17, 9:00 a.m.: "Henda, look what just came over the radiology wires!"

One week after my phone call to my representative, I was prepped and ready to be taken to the OR for my lumpectomy to remove the tumor. My radiologist rushed into my room. She handed me a printout with the news. Connecticut had just passed a bill to inform women about dense breast tissue—the first state in the nation to pass such legislation. I took it as a great omen that my own effort in Texas might not be a futile attempt after all!

After much debate my medical team decided to remove the

tumor right away. Although the tumor was large, my surgeon felt confident that she would be able to save my breast. In the first of many decisions I opted out of a double mastectomy. My BRACA gene testing was negative; I didn't carry the breast cancer gene mutation. Not ready to lose my breasts, I chose less invasive surgery. My surgeon also removed my first four sentinel lymph nodes to be examined by the pathologist. If cancer cells were present, all my lymph nodes in my right arm would have to be removed.

Barely a month since my diagnosis, breast cancer was quickly shaping me into a different person. It forced me onto a road where I could see the path but had little knowledge where the way led. I could not have predicted the significant lessons that were waiting.

June 27, 2:30 p.m.: "Sweeties . . . darling bunnies . . . something happened while you were at camp. I got breast cancer."

My cancer diagnosis occurred the week before my kids left for their annual two-week summer camp in the piney woods of East Texas. I was unwilling to send them off to camp with such devastating information. I didn't say a word and had my first surgery while they happily enjoyed the bliss of being carefree kids.

I blurted out my newsflash to the camp directors when we picked them up. By then the tear tracks were well formed down my cheeks. With a bandaged breast I had no idea how to confess my tumor secrets to my most precious ones. I felt so guilty that I'd withheld the information from them and distressed that they might feel I didn't trust them enough to share. After we exhausted all their camp stories, I finally announced my un-fun update. I had read several books the week before on how to tell your kids you had cancer. But in the moment I just wished that I never had to peel their childhood innocence away. I could tolerate the demands of a breast cancer diagnosis, but it saddened me to be their teacher on this subject of survival.

I held my breath for their response. My ten-year-old son cut to the chase and asked me if I would die. I honestly had to confess that I didn't know. He next questioned what would kill me faster, poison or cancer? Content that I wasn't dropping dead from poison soon, he continued to read his book. My eight-year-old daughter asked if I lost my hair, could I get a wig that looked like her dirty blonde hair? Yeah! No brainer, cherished girl!

The rest of the way home I watched the East Texas countryside pass by, recalling the awe I felt when my firstborn, Mateo, grew in my body. Feeling him move, hearing his steady heartbeat, seeing him on the sonogram screen, and carrying his blurry black-and-white screenshot to show off to everybody. His birth was a small miracle on a very icy December day in 1998 when I held him in my arms. He was just six pounds, three ounces with a head of golden hair—my little love bug.

The wonder repeated itself with my daughter, Dominique,

twenty-four months later. Her January birthday was sunny and bright, and she allowed me to have a well-planned delivery day down to a great pedicure beforehand. When I held her moments after her birth, she quenched her thirst from my breasts for more than an hour before she was ready to greet the day. That's my girl—it's not necessary to face anything hungry.

My efforts to teach them independence and resourcefulness started when they were born. It had been hard to watch them stumble so they could learn to get back up. I often had to fight the urge to shelter them, but I knew the importance of learning the art of resilience. I encouraged them to pursue their goals, to be the best they could be, and to seek out what inspired them wholeheartedly. Looking back I suspect it was my calling as their mother from the start. Was I to show them by example what fighting back was all about? Demonstrate how to overcome our biggest challenges? Teach them how to never give up?

Unfortunately I required a second lumpectomy within weeks of my first surgery. It was to ensure that I had what is called "clear margins"—2mm of tissue surrounding the tumor without any cancer cells present. But the enormous homerun I scored? They added me to the radiology case studies because my initial MRI was indeed wrong! Although I had a small cluster of cancer cells in my first lymph node, the next three nodes were clear, allowing me to keep the rest of my lymph nodes. Hell yes! My first of many lucky breaks! And this time my kids were by my side in the hospital.

The following summer when I dropped them off at camp, their hugs proved to be a little tighter around my neck, and my son whispered in my ear, "Mama, please don't let anything happen to you while we are gone!"

One Traveling Bandaged Dense Breast, Late July 2009

DESPERATE TO CLING TO some semblance of normalcy after my diagnosis, (but totally against my doctor's orders), I charged ahead with our plans to spend a two-week summer vacation in Peru. Trekking with the family from the Amazon rainforest to Machu Picchu, Cusco, and the Sacred Valley while recovering from two recent surgeries was dumb. Okay. Plain stupid. Toward the end of our vacation we found ourselves at Lake Titicaca, the highest navigational lake in the world at 15,400 feet. Legend considers it the birthplace of the Inca.

That morning I had my coca leaves read by an old Inca shaman who of course raved about all my good fortune and happiness. He promised that my leaves showed a long life. Uh huh? His smile was too wide for me to tell him about the big "C." Who could tell the future anyway? Maybe he and the leaves were right. Days later from inside an ICU, I would want to ask for a complete refund. Or else some fresh leaves!

On the way to Arequipa, the White City, I had a strange sensation in my chest as if a gorilla were slowly sitting down on me. Each intake of air was a painful exercise of my lungs expanding and collapsing. However, I kept this to myself, thinking that a lower altitude would solve the problem. Besides, Arequipa was our last stop and the birthplace of my father-in-law. I didn't want to ruin the highlight of the trip for my children to see where Grandpa was from.

Our sprawling hotel was located on a river near downtown built in the signature white volcanic stone of the city. But by bedtime I felt lousy, and my breathing difficulty had worsened.

August 1, 9:00 a.m.: "Tu corazón . . . medio es muerto." Half of your heart is dead.

¡¿Qué?! Comeagain? I had no doubt that the Peruvian cardiologist standing in front of me was a madman. Only someone insane could utter those words. Me? A heart attack? *Crazy old man!* He rattled on in fast Spanish, way above my basic conversational level, as my mind strained to recall how I had gotten there.

I had woken up that morning at 5:00 a.m. with a rubber tube clasping my lungs in a vise grip. I couldn't breathe, my arms and hands were numb, and I was vomiting. I left my husband behind with our sleeping kids in our hotel room and walked out into the deserted early morning city streets to flag a cab. The Clinica Arequipa was the only private hospital for a tourist like me. In my limited Spanish I instructed the cab driver to head there *"muy rapido!"* I sensed that something was very wrong, but I was optimistic that simply inhaling forced oxygen would restore the struggle of taking a breath. Only later did I realize how dismal my symptoms were.

When I arrived at the hospital I quickly found myself caught in the worst nightmare imaginable. But it was no dream. Instead I was trapped on a very narrow metal cot in the middle of Peru. I had a bunch of needles stuck in my arms and an oxygen mask covered my face. A frantic group of nurses and doctors swarmed around me and I desperately desired for my Spanish to be better.

The cardiologist left after blurting out the status about my half-dead heart. I had an urgent need to escape from there and reached for my cell phone to call my husband . . . only to find that I had no service! In my haste to catch a cab I had also left the hotel name and number behind. A young intern who spoke English finally came to my aid and offered to find my family. Based on my very vague description of the hotel, he pieced it together and reached Rick. I begged him to hurry to the clinic and could only trust that I would stay alive until he and my kids found me. In the aftermath of a cancer diagnosis, dying in a hallway in Peru was completely unscripted.

My body had been poked and probed the entire summer by my cancer doctors in Dallas. They would surely have picked up on any heart defects? I was careful not to elaborate to anyone about my still- bandaged right breast. There was no reason to heighten the freak-out factor and complicate their focus.

Filled with apprehension, I took the hand of my Peruvian intern and asked, "If I were your sister, what would you suggest I do?" Without hesitation he urged me to be admitted to their ICU and be treated for a heart attack. He reminded me that the EKG clearly showed the event and the cardiac enzyme blood tests confirmed the diagnosis. The longer I stalled, the less chance there was to reverse long-term damage, much less save me from dying. Out of options and stuck in a *Twilight Zone* episode straight from a Halloween special to boost Nielsen ratings, I agreed.

My family's shocked faces mirrored my own when they walked into the makeshift ER a little later. I felt as if all of creation had sucker- punched me hard with some sneaky bitch moves. In the intensive care I was shot full of mystery medicines, swallowed pills without names, and had IV fluids pumped into me. My basic Spanish served no purpose, and I fully surrendered to my caregivers. Their mission was to make sure I didn't die on their watch.

Suddenly breast cancer didn't seem like such a bad deal. At

least I could say my goodbyes in an organized way compared to my heart stopping with its very next beat. A vice of sheer panic over my own death clenched me very tightly. I had never been this scared. Ever. I felt lost to my core. The ICU nurse dutifully sat next to my bed while monitoring the machines I was hooked up to. Oh, said machines and ICU were straight from a 1950s movie set! Let's just say that the ICU lacked the glamour and gloss of modern technology. Her English was absent, and I didn't have the energy to try to practice my Spanish. My family stopped by a couple of times a day. But for the most part I was left to drown inside my own mind. I was catapulted back to the hell of June 10 when I didn't think my night could be darker. Only this time I felt myself slipping off the slope out of reach of any shreds I could grab.

Through the small window in my hospital room I could see the El Misti volcano. El Misti is the middle volcano of the three circling Arequipa—the only one still active and holding its place on the Ring of Fire outlining the Pacific tectonic plate. At 19,100 feet its impressive, symmetrical snowcapped peak flirted with me. Out of options about how else to save myself, I made a deal with a volcano, vowing that I would one day stand on its summit. If I survived this ordeal at all.

After three days I was finally considered stable enough for the old cardiologist in charge to clear me to travel to Lima to see a second cardiologist—one who could speak English and was a

fellow of the American College of Cardiology. Finally we were
cooking with gas! Hallelujah! He alerted the airline, and I flew
to Lima in a wheelchair

carrying travel permission papers although I had no idea what
they said. "Okay, whatever—just get me to Dallas!" I prayed. The
Lima doc then blessed my transfer home if Rick would give me
anti- coagulant shots in my stomach and I would take about ten
tablets every four hours. Okay, whatever!

I finally arrived in Dallas two days later—still in a wheelchair
and shaking like a ragdoll. We went straight to UT Southwestern.
In addition to the breast cancer department, I became fast friends
with the cardiology unit. After a string of tests including a heart
catheterization, my cardiologist changed the Peruvian doomsday
diagnosis to pericarditis—an inflammation of my heart lining. In
other words I had just been caught in the perfect storm of wrong
place at the wrong time. "Your heart is healthy and strong," he
assured me. Alrighty, then! Let the believing begin!

Before my own *Grey's Anatomy* drama-filled episode, our
Peruvian excursion had taken us into the dense Amazon
rainforest to one of its tributaries. There I bought a simple, hand-
carved bracelet for two dollars from another old Inca man while
visiting his primitive hut and learning about their customs. It was
made from coconut shell and had a woven pattern in the center
that reminded me of a spider web. The man used very thin strips
of cornhusks to create the pattern, which have slowly unraveled

over time. I seldom wear it because it has become very delicate. However, whenever it graces my wrist, it reminds me how fragile our lives are.

Aside from the myocardial infarction (that sounds so much better than a heart attack!), Peru silently initiated me into a love affair with seven great wonders of the world. Our tie would span the next seven years on my own path of discovery and healing. After the Amazon, the Sacred Valley was our next stop. Sunrise over Machu Picchu debuted the first wonder. Steeped in sanctity and surrounded by mountains bigger than any manmade phenomenon, I reveled in how the sun slowly bathed the age-old ruins in light. And how the mountains leisurely shed their deep purple nightgown for a bright day coat. According to Inca moral code, *Ama suwa, ama llulla, ama quella,* one should not steal, tell any lies, or be lazy. In this sacred place in the Andes, my spirit awakened to strive to live by my own newfound moral code: authentic, vulnerable, and worthy.

But first I had to find the strength in the coming weeks to scale two very large mountains: cardiac rehab and breast radiation. Surprisingly, the universe was also about to upgrade the script from just a B-movie without consulting me first. I was the leading unpaid female in this drama after all!

My Not-So-Finest Hour Eating Darn Fine BBQ!

I HAVE A LARGE hourglass filled with fine white sand. It sits in my living room on a table that was hand carved from a cypress tree near Caddo Lake in East Texas. Every time I pass by it I flip the glass over and allow the sand to trickle through the thin center separating the two delicate bubbles. Occasionally the sand gets stuck, and I must shake the glass for it to drop. I enjoy watching its passage and find satisfaction that I can invert it repeatedly, unlike the ability to reverse events from my past.

My warped sense of humor called for creating a T-shirt to commemorate my 2009 incidents thus far. I thought of

"Survived. Despite the market crash." Or how about "Breast Cancer? Heart Attack? Got it!" Or maybe "Held together by spit and duct tape."

My breast cancer radiation treatments had to be delayed while I focused on restoring my heart's full function. Initially I was slated for a twelve-week program at a cardiac rehabilitation complex in Dallas. Reminiscent of the waiting room after my cancer diagnosis, I was the odd one yet again. My companions were grey-haired aging men recovering from stents and bypasses. Together we wore our heart monitors and worked out under the watchful eyes of the nurses and cardiologist on duty. All of us were absolutely committed to the same end goal: a healthy heart.

Fear was my confidante and clung to me. My days evolved into a sick mind game of "which was worse?" Rogue cancer cells growing post-surgery or half a heart? I often caught my fingers on my carotid artery. Instead of counting the beats I would chant with each one "I'm alive, I'm alive, I'm alive." I knew firsthand that when the beat stopped my life would end. It was a reality that I could not swap for the innocence of the clichés about existing in the moment. I had always understood they were true, but I didn't really know how true until we became blood brothers and they crawled into the very fiber of my being.

After four weeks my cardiologist pronounced my heart well and my rehab finished. Easy for him to say! Being OCD came with benefits. I bought a hospital-grade blood pressure machine and monitored my heart at least seven times a day. Imagine a spreadsheet with many rows and columns filled with daily blood pressure data for weeks and months. Now imagine my cardiologist on the receiving end of such information regularly. You really should add him to your holiday mailing list. He is a great man!

Breast radiation followed immediately after my rehab. I was beat up and fed up with all things medicine, and the thought of what was ahead loomed like endless steamy summer days in hell. To start, the target area had to be carefully mapped. The radiation oncologist marked up my right breast and chest with dots and dashes using a black marker to align with the radiation machine's beams. They covered the marks with clear stickers and instructed me to make sure that the stickers stayed put and dry for the duration of treatment. Alternatively, I could opt for permanent tattoos across my skin. Eeewww, where do I check the "No Thank You" box? There was no need to turn this into forever anything! Seriously, I would rather have tattooed "I love Rufus" on my bicep than to get my chest radiation marks inked!

They then created a custom mold of my upper body to help me stay in the same position. This aided the accuracy of the beam to pass through my body whilst destroying good and bad cells. Arms raised above my head, I lay on my back as the warm blue fluid in the plastic bag underneath me took the shape of my torso and arms. Afterward they added my name to it, and I was curious whether they might offer it to me as a souvenir at the end.

The traditional radiation protocol called for thirty-six days of treatment, but luckily (and thankfully) I qualified for a shorter, far more concentrated exposure. My last day of treatment was October 2, 2009. By that time my skin was burned from the inside out and peeling badly. It was like having a severe sunburn within every cell inside my body. I was emotionally falling apart and holding on to a very flimsy thread of faith. Time and again, even in my darkest of days, sunlight always looked for a crack to filter through. I just had to keep believing in that single ray of light.

The caution signage on the door to the radiation chamber reminded me of a scene from a science fiction horror flick. For sixteen days I walked through the door. I lay down on a narrow table underneath the radiation machine, removed my arms from my hospital gown sleeves, and rested into my "Henda" mold. Next the staff aligned the marks and dots with the beast's laser beams. During the next ten minutes the monster machine rotated around my body. It made clicking and whirring sounds like some alien licking its chops before it devoured me. I could never stop my tears flowing down my cheeks in little wet streams. They pooled together in the hollows of my collarbones and formed little eddies that spilled over the edge. How I detested every single one of those sixteen days.

My radiation appointment was every day at 9:00 a.m. sharp.

Afterward I walked to one of the oldest barbeque joints in Dallas— the original Sonny Bryan's on Inwood Road across from UT Southwestern. I was usually one of the first customers of the day and ordered a side of coleslaw, two colossal onion rings, and either the pork ribs or slow-smoked brisket. I would slide into one of the snug vintage school desks all lined up in a row and drizzle the warm barbeque sauce over my plate. Although there was no relief from the painful sunburn inside my body, the food brought me comfort and allowed me to briefly rearrange my scattered thoughts. Only years later did I question what my heart was thinking about the daily post- radiation cholesterol pile-up on a plate.

When Lightning Strikes

Crossing the street from my latest nightmare at the hospital allowed me to face my older ones more graciously.

My BBQ lunchtime reflections brought me back to the months just prior to my breast cancer diagnosis in June 2009. That spring, before terrible luck and illness altered my fate, depression had swept over me with the unexpected speed and ferocity of a tsunami. I was reluctant to replay those days. But it was as if the scorching heat from the radiation in my chest wanted to ignite my whole being. Its intensity compelled me to re-traverse my old *Way of Sorrows*.

How will I kill myself? It was the most frightening thought that had ever entered my mind. But there it was on a fateful day in mid- February 2009. I was driving down the Dallas North Tollway back to downtown after showing houses in a suburb. I didn't start with asking myself *if* I could commit suicide; instead I contemplated *how*. Knowing myself well, I recognized that my choice of self-destruction would somehow involve my beloved ocean and scuba diving.

My infatuation with scuba diving had begun the week after I arrived in the United States in 1990. Almost 300 dives later, the ocean blue is well acquainted with my issues. It understands how I first float at the surface to let my claustrophobia exhale and breathe. When at ease I can submit to descending into its vastness and discover the gems awaiting me. How magnificent they always are! I've been enveloped in the wings of a stingray, grabbed by a giant octopus's suction cups, and entertained by wild dolphin frolicking.

Humpback whales serenaded me with their complex and haunting songs, indisputably one of the most profound compositions of sound I ever listened to. Cave diving got checked off the list. Once, and only once, did I sink into a cave with hundreds of feet of solid rock above my head. Despite being a self-proclaimed "badass," my bravado evaporated fast when I squeezed myself and my scuba tank through the narrow passages of several underwater tunnels.

Unlike the sinister realm of cave diving, my most favored dive site is a cliff dive, also known as a wall dive. Not only do these locations teem with colorful reef fish, but you can also find large pelagic fish like sharks, rays, jacks, and groupers. My favorite underwater symphony is the melody of my own bubbles mixed with the infinite chatter of fish feeding on the reef. Covered in abundant coral growing vertically on the steep overhangs, the wall can suddenly plunge into the ocean's depth.

While suspended against a wall without any seabed as a barrier, paying attention to one's depth is paramount. Currents can easily sweep you into eternity, particularly if the intent is to never return to the surface anyway. This was my poison of choice. Being a seasoned diver I realized at some point I would become delirious from the nitrogen floating in my blood. In dive slang, the effects of nitrogen narcosis are like one martini for every thirty-three feet of descent. Having dived already to 142 feet in the Blue Hole in Belize on a past dive trip, and following the hypothetical "Martini Law," I figured I would require about five stiff drinks or 165 feet to reach oblivion. My impairment would increase as my depth escalated, and I would slowly lose my judgment to ascend to a shallower depth. The nitrogen narcosis would relieve all anxiety, and instead I would face complete serenity. The selection of my final wall dive would be based on its brilliance. Both in the abundance of marine creatures big and small, as well as its dramatic drops and cobalt blue waters filtering the sun rays to wash the coral reefs into a blooming summer garden.

I was horrified by my thoughts. Contemplating the madness of ending it all was the most foreign place I had ever ventured inside my own mind. I had already lived several lifetimes of overcoming obstacles—quitting on myself should have been unimaginable. How did I get to this desperately lonely place? But more important, how the hell would I get out? Truthfully, I was clueless how to ask for help in one of my blackest hours. I pulled off the highway into a fast food parking lot and sobbed uncontrollably. Despite having a lot of friends, who could I call with this dilemma? It was as if my guardian angels comprehended that it was time for them to intrude fast with a godly intervention.

I dialed Sam. We had not talked in a while, and he seldom answered calls. Miraculously, he picked up on the second ring. I must have sounded worse than I felt as he invited me to come and meet him at White Rock Lake. We sat for a while outside talking on the steps of the old Filter building next to the rowing boathouse. I shared with him the depth of my unhappiness in my marriage, the piercing pain of being caught up in a place I felt like an alien, and the agony of being the most unauthentic person I knew. I finally had the courage to confess that my ongoing project of reinventing "Henda" had gone horribly wrong.

His kindness and wisdom were raindrops falling on my thirsty presence. When I left there I felt I was tossed a life preserver. I had a plan that didn't include a wall dive to eternity. Oh, how thin is that edge between sanity and stir crazy! How narrow that ledge we tread daily. How dark our demons when they are hidden and therefore in charge.

Sam's plan was simple: get me fit. At the time, I felt like (and looked like) a beached baby humpback whale. I weighed almost twenty-five pounds more than my ideal weight today. Being short and small boned does not allow me to hide any pounds in my pockets. I had no muscle definition, and my thighs and upper arms had the familiar jiggle of dimpled cellulite. I can use many excuses as to why and how I'd allowed myself to arrive at the gates of self-loathing. But ultimately it's quite simple. When you avoid your own eyes long enough in the mirror while brushing your teeth daily, you should anticipate self-destruction in some form. My time bomb triggered in 1990 when I boarded the plane to the US and pretended that I was an orphan. Nicky's death in 2006 lit the fuse that led to my winter's depression and the 2009 explosion.

When I'd contemplated how to end it all in February 2009, I had no idea that only a few months later all my guardian angels would quit their jobs. Seriously, how could they let me have breast cancer and a heart attack back to back? After all we had been through together growing up? I'm still mad at them. I needed a serious course correction, but between them, God, the universe, and all the other divine bodies, did they not check in with each other? Or maybe they did. Whatever the case, the strategy worked. Grandly. I'm quite confident they are all smiling fondly down on me these days!

In a cosmic sense of good timing, I hit rock bottom *before* my two-for-one special. My brush with death jumpstarted my ascent. In diving terms I had essentially reached an "out of air emergency" in February. When you are in deep water and out of air, diver protocol requires that you drop your weights, spread your arms and legs to slow your ascent, and continuously exhale, making an *ahhhh* sound until you reach the surface. Getting to the top, however, is the first of your problems. Your lungs could explode; you can burst all sorts of vessels in your brain. But at least you might make it out alive!

The Stink of Fear

I N MY LAST DAY of radiation I celebrated the finale of torture with a portion of ribs and brisket and a full order of Sonny Bryan's famous onion rings. I was an affirmed mess and very unsure of where to navigate next. I felt betrayed by my very being. The burden to somehow hold it together for my kids and husband was almost unbearable.

In the following weeks it took all my self-control not to just start screaming when friendly grocery checkout clerks asked, "How're you doing today?" My enthusiasm for my real estate career also faded fast. Who cared about selling houses when your heart was about to stop? I felt like a preprogrammed robot each morning: shower, dress, feed the kids, do the laundry, show houses, sell houses, shop for groceries, smile, smile, and smile. (Yelling, shouting, and screaming were not algorithms allowed in the code.)

The intensity of my despair drove me to see a therapist. Referred by a friend, she specialized in post-traumatic stress. I learned what F.E.A.R. stands for—False Evidence Appearing Real. Having never suffered from anxiety I became an expert in another subject quickly.

It was paralyzing. I obsessed about my heart beating and panicked at the very thought of it not beating. My cardiologist let me carry a portable ECG for a month. Every time I felt like I was having a heart attack, the compact electrocardiogram would transmit my heart's reading to a 24-hour monitoring center. Countless times during the day you could find me pulled off on the side of the road with the little device feverishly pressed against my left breast.

The radiation sunburn took a while to heal. My disfigured right breast was a constant reminder that my road to cancer remission was in its infancy. As I imagined cancer cells multiplying throughout my body, I was once again immobilized with the terror of believing that I would be a casualty of the disease. The depth of my anxiety left me powerless. I dreaded waking each day. And my nightly angst when going to bed drove me into the arms of sleeping pills. I felt like such a loser. A quitter. A failure. Half dead, I thought I might as well drop dead.

The therapist encouraged me to treat my terror like a toddler. I could not ignore it. Instead I should give it the attention it was seeking. It was a great analogy because I clearly remembered when my two children had their two-year-old moments of lying flat on their tummies in the grocery aisle while screaming blue murder. Meanwhile I pretended that I lived on one of the shelves and had no idea whose kids they were. *Where was their mom? I mean, really, could she not control her kids?*

How do you pull your ass out of these kinds of thorny thickets? I wasn't sure. Ms. Therapist wanted me to "validate my emotions" and stop thinking that they didn't fit my persona. (Easy for her to say!) She kept telling me that my distress was a "wave I should ride to shore." (Pity I only learned to surf years later!) Ugh, and then we had Step Three. Totally out of reach. Like a balloon that slipped your grasp on its way to the stratosphere. "Be kind to Henda" and "don't chastise yourself for being weak." (But I was brilliant at beating up on myself!) Vulnerability was a foreign place I had seldom visited. Nope. Grit and defenseless were incompatible words never used together in my sentences. How could those guardian angels set me up like this?! I was three years old again and scared every day. Not just of the dark and cockroaches. I was terrified of dying. I came face to face with the young me—the one who had thought she wouldn't survive either. In a surprising convergence of then and now, I faced the irony of dealing in my own life's currency. The little warrior meeting the old one. My singular quest to just keep breathing made the old crusades against my mother and finding my father appear so infinitely small. My psyche was back in front of the Leadwood tree again seeking guidance—only this time stripped several more layers bare. Without faith or strength I was inexperienced in how to move forward.

The Accidental Making of a Lobbyist

W HILE I WAS LOST in the woods, my state representative, Allen Vaught, was slowly gathering support for the breast density bill that I had begged him to help me author. I certainly was not in any condition to focus on learning political prowess. It was up to him to solidify the right army of supporters. The state of Texas has a legislative session every two years, from approximately January to June. Since the 2009 session was over by that point, we had about a year to prepare to file a bill with the Texas legislature in Austin in January 2011.

In the late fall of 2009 I decided that another excursion to South Africa would brighten my drab and gloomy outlook. Maybe my South African friends could help me practice my latest endeavor of being nice to myself. It was difficult to think my mood could sink any lower, and the thought of spending time in the African bush was very comforting.

The week before my departure I played a card game called Texas Hold 'Em in a charity poker tournament for a local cause. If you are a good card player you don't want me at your table. My decisions are irrational. I fold when I should hold, bluff when I should fold, and generally go all-in when my fate depends on the "river." (The river is the dealer's last card.) I live and die on the river, darling! It either gets me a seat at the final table or a very early night.

On this night fate intervened once again and caused my elimination early on. I found myself next to another doomed player, watching the final ten players duke it out for the big screen TV as first prize. How surprising when I learned he was a seasoned senior lobbyist for a very large national organization. Really? What a coincidence.

I quickly filled him in on the breast density bill and my aspirations to change the standard of care. He tried hard not to burst my bubble, but he was also honest about the political process in Austin. Although my efforts were admirable, he cautioned me not to get my hopes up. In a very kind way, Douglas basically told me that hell would freeze before a highly divided Texas senate and house would pass a breast cancer bill during the first session it was filed. Really? Douglas didn't yet understand that "It's not possible" are words that I thrive on. Additionally, with my insane fright of death, I simply didn't have time to go back for a second or third session. Time was of the essence! Seeking as much free advice as possible, I speculated aloud how does one pass a bill. Hypothetically speaking of course, but how *does* one pass a bill in one session having had no experience and no money to pay a contract lobbyist? Simple, he said. Buy the book The *Midwest Academy*, study it from cover to cover, and implement each step while lobbying every noteworthy player in Austin. By that he meant the state representatives and their staff, the state senators and all their staff, all the lobbyists for all the major medical groups like the American Cancer Society, the Texas Hospital Association, and the Texas Radiology Society, and every other prominent player that would care about a healthcare bill, which is *everybody*. Learn all their names, he continued, the issues they care about, and try to find a connection so they will give you two minutes for your readymade elevator speech.

Okey dokey! Let's start by begging for Douglas's business card. Intrigued, I also asked what this remarkable book was about. He explained that it teaches the methods and skills to enable ordinary people to actively participate in the democratic process and effectively organize for social justice and change. The day before my flight to Johannesburg, we located the book at a Dallas public library and my husband kindly picked it up. Holy crap! It was enormous! I ended up reading the book cover to cover twice during my two sixteen-hour flights to and from Johannesburg. I reread it during the days while on safari in the bush. In fact it was the only thing that I read during my entire trip. I felt confident afterward that I could pass a multiple-choice exam with extended essays, if quizzed.

Armed with part one of my free advice, I felt comfortable that with Allen Vaught's guidance I could politic my way through Austin. I had a pair of cowboy boots, a blingy belt buckle, and jeans and had also gained a decent ability to dance the Texas two-step and the more progressive triple-step . . . with variations and twirling, might I say. (Really. I'm not lying.) I naively felt that my untrained, unelected, and clueless status would work in my favor. Of course I was marked to fail before I ever started. Just like when I was young. But the underdog and I were old friends at this point. Underestimating me has always worked in my favor and has been my coat rack and umbrella stand in my foyer for half a lifetime.

Meanwhile, radiation had turned my tissues, muscles, and skin into scrambled eggs and ended my rowing. I missed how the rhythm of my oars would carve at the water like a sculptor patiently revealing his creation from stone. While rowing I often found comfort in buckets of sunlight gold across White Rock Lake in the early mornings or occasionally at night. In addition to gold, sometimes I was treated to blood-red stains on the water. Both enveloped me in brief moments of perfect peace. How I longed for those times.

Before my eyes, the last of my rowing muscles vanished as 2009 was ending. Although still slender, I didn't do much exercise past June (understandably, I might add). By December I was worried that my fat clothes I'd stuck in the attic might make a comeback. Luckily my anxiety disorder didn't drive me to food! I was so ready to see the last of this year. For Halloween I dressed as a warrior princess. I guess only I saw the humor in my useless plastic sword—a symbol of how beaten and disarmed I felt on the inside. I could totally visualize me being on my knees, sword against my chest. Okay, high drama, but bear with me . . . the year was almost done. Had I suspected then what was in store for me, I would have fallen on that imaginary sword!

AfterShock

THE UNITED STATES GENERAL elections of 2010 unfolded upstairs on my laptop and the 11.5-hour time difference made it still very early in Dallas. The voting polls had only been open a few hours when I turned the light out to try to sleep some before the results were announced.

While I trained for the race during the summer and fall of 2010, my state congressman, Allen Vaught, met with many doctors across Texas from UT Southwestern, Baylor Medical Center, and the Paul L. Foster School of Medicine in El Paso to the M.D. Anderson Cancer Center in Houston. He sought their support for legislation he planned to introduce during the 2011 Texas legislative session. The bill would require FDA-approved mammogram facilities to inform women about dense breast tissue and the limitations of a mammogram detecting a tumor in dense breasts. The legislation would also ensure that at-risk women had access to supplemental screening.

I had one more week left in India and the next morning, just before I left for the airport to catch my flight to Varanasi, I was almost too anxious to log on to my computer. Vaught, a moderate Democrat, had served two terms and his challenger was a newcomer Tea Party Republican. I was shocked when I saw the final results. Vaught had lost the reelection. I was speechless. Devastated. Angry. Unspeakably disappointed. Bloody angry. Dumbstruck. Crushed. Nooooooooo!

Darn it! I didn't have a Plan B. He had to win. That was the plan! The bottom dropped out of my stomach and I thought I was going to vomit. My ears were ringing and I could see little black spots in front of me. I had to sit down on the bed to prevent myself from falling. How could chance play this sick trick on me after all that had happened? It wasn't possible that my aspiration to save a few lives had become a distant mirage fading fast into obscurity. Over the past twenty-four hours I had caught the thermals, soared, but then crashed into pieces.

I made peace with the fact that my ambition to change the standard of care for women with dense breast tissue might have to be shelved, barring mythical intervention. I still had complete faith that my cancer had a purpose. I would just have to let each day reveal what that looked like. Governor Perry would simply have to sign a law during the next session that neither he nor anybody in Austin had any knowledge about. Although maybe not religious in the traditional sense, I undoubtedly believed in miracles. C'mon, divine ones, pay attention!

There is special providence in the fall
of a sparrow. If it be now,
'tis not to come; if it be not to come,
it will be now; if it be not
now, yet it will come—the readiness is all. Since no man, of
aught he leaves, knows what is't to leave betimes? Let be.

—SHAKESPEARE, *HAMLET*, ACT 5, SCENE 2

Charging Hell with a Bucket of Ice Water

I SAT ON A bench inside the Texas capitol in Austin trying to interpret the map that showed the different legislative offices. I might as well have been studying an ancient treasure map in Greek. I felt quite teary and had no doubt that if I was on a reality game show I would be voted off. The capitol was a maze, and I had no foggy idea how to locate the representatives and senators' offices where I was supposed to be in less than ten minutes.

Just hours before, on a very crisp Tuesday morning in late January 2011, I had my first introduction with this iconic Texas landmark. The pale pink granite of the capitol was washed in the warm rays of the early morning sun. Atop the dome Lady Liberty silently observed my approach and I felt sure that the same thought had crossed both our minds: "What the heck is *she* doing here?"

My stomach was a tight knot of nerves. It was a complete miracle for me to be in Austin. I had given up expectations that anything could be accomplished after Vaught lost his reelection bid in November. But the mysterious twists and turns of my cancer train were not slowing down. A Texas representative from Houston ended up hiring Vaught's legislative director who then presented my bill to her new boss, who also happened to be firmly committed to women's health issues. Suddenly we had a real bill to pass! My latest ally was in her second term, and I easily promised her my full support to help in any way possible.

I found myself in Austin at the start of the New Year because my dense breast tissue bill named "Henda's Law" was being filed in the 82nd legislative session in the state of Texas's house and senate. The sponsored senator and state representative had invited me to attend what was for them a routine activity, whereas for me it had altered my world's spin.

Mentally putting on my big girl panties, I got up from the bench, stepped through the capitol building's wooden doors, and went into the rotunda. Surrounded by portraits of the past presidents of the Republic of Texas and the past governors of the state of Texas, the enormity of the moment caught me by surprise. September 2003's memory was still fresh when I took the oath to become an American citizen and recited my first Pledge of Allegiance.

Eight short years later I was now witness to a bill carrying my name being filed at the Texas state capitol to help women fight breast cancer. Geez, Louise. Not sure who did the choosing here as I had neither a hat nor cattle to fit into this party.

"Breathe, just breathe," I kept repeating to myself. "And please don't cry . . . or throw up!" My tears had a mind of their own and forced themselves past all the naysayers. It had been less than two years since I was knocked sideways by cancer. I had a strange sense that I stood exactly where I was supposed to be at that moment. Without sounding corny, I felt inherently responsible to help other women avoid a late diagnosis.

Sigh. India had certainly sorted some of my "psychological issues" regarding my heart but I was still a nutcase at large. Not to worry. I'm better these days, although I cry even easier! But don't you agree that it seemed predetermined? Like cancer handpicked me? I think the plan always was to transport me from South Africa to Austin. Anyway, it makes me feel better thinking that the whole C-thing was part of a higher purpose.

I finally located the senator's office. He was one of the senior members, a longtime legislator and a Democrat. His stern farewell message matched his imposing stature as he towered over me. "Little girl, although I filed the senate bill, it's up to you to garner bipartisan support to get it passed!"

Sufficiently warned, my second stop was the capitol gift store to buy the 2011 legislature handbook. Inside were all the senators and representatives' names listed, their office locations, as well as their legislative directors and aides. I also bought a striking Texas star bracelet with ten vermeil gold stars linked together. It was for good luck. My promise? I would not take it off until the bill had passed.

The size of the capitol from the outside is completely misleading, as half of it is underground. Juggling the advice in the handbook and the information on my map was like trying to scale a massive mountain in flip-flops. Paging through the handbook, I realized I had no idea how to implement the advice from my fall reading, *The Midwest Academy*. On a whim I decided to initially target the state representatives from the North Texas area, but my attempts to speak to anybody misfired. I never made it past the secretaries safeguarding their domains. I soon found myself on another bench ready to shed more tears. I could hear Mandela whisper, "Courage is not the absence of fear, but the triumph over it. The brave man is not he who does not feel afraid, but he who conquers that fear." I knew he would advise me to implement a better plan than my current Wonderful World of Waterworks. But until then I felt like a complete crying loser.

Searching for a Whisper in a Whirlwind

FORTUNATELY, MY FRIEND TRACEY lived nearby and just like so much else, meeting her in India during the Himalayan 100 race had proved to be no coincidence. She was my hut mate on the race at 13,000 feet and my steadfast companion on the painful Day Four when finishing seemed unlikely. I was equally bruised and battered after my first day as a lobbyist when I arrived on her doorstep in Austin. Having a friend that evening was like a cold glass of lemonade on a blazing Texas summer day. Staying with her would be a godsend in the weeks and months to come, along with her support, encouragement, and friendship.

The next morning, armed with photocopies of the bill and dressed in a dark pink dress given to me by Tracey, I was invigorated to try once more. I almost felt like waving to Lady Liberty this time as I walked up to the daunting pink granite structure. Almost immediately I ran into an aide for a very senior house representative. He was familiar with my efforts, thanks to our mutual lobbyist friend, Douglas. I told him about my struggles to get my foot in the door the day before, and he gave some advice that became one of the jewels inside my Austin war chest. He coached me to hand out something tangible that would stand out on desks brimming over with paperwork from the thousands of bills filed each session. Additionally, he counseled me to have a very short, memorable summary of the bill as part of my handout with the "what" and "why" very prominently displayed. His parting suggestion was to have a pitch-perfect elevator speech at the ready.

I decided to spend the rest of that day just getting lost inside the maze. It was like a scavenger hunt. I randomly picked an office from my handbook and tried to find it without walking in too many circles. Once I figured out that the letters N, S, W, or E in front of the room numbers represented directions on a compass, I was in good shape. And here you thought I joked about my sincere failure at understanding directions!

When I left the capitol at the end of the day, I blew a kiss to my statue friend perched high above. Bravely, young leaves had burst early from their sleepy cocoon to defy the late winter setting. The air smelled of earth and freshness, and I envisioned bottling its distinct fragrance. It was my kind of season. I could not help but sense a resurgence of hope that maybe my efforts would not be a complete fiasco.

Driving north back home to Dallas, I had no idea how many times I would undertake this same 400-mile round trip to the state house in the coming months. My first introduction to the reality of politics felt like an old-school hazing. It dawned on me that instead of trying to become a politician, I should stick with what I was familiar with. Sales. I was no politician and had no skill passing a law. But I knew how to sell. I had been a top residential real estate expert selling a lot of high-end homes. By the time I pulled into my driveway that evening it was suddenly so clear—passing this bill would require me to perform the best sales job ever!

Anticipating that I would be back in Austin very soon, I had little time to get professionally made handouts, so I went the homemade route. I had learned something else from trying to get past the secretaries. Not only is "dense breast tissue" a tongue twister, but people's eyes quickly glazed over. The regular response of "Wait, what?" after my elevator speech was almost comical. There was never enough time to explain what the three words meant. The perfect "show" was a picture of my own mammogram hiding a four -centimeter tumor. Almost poetically, just prior to my breast surgery in 2009, the radiologist had implanted a very tiny titanium ribbon to mark my tumor location—an image that showed up clearly on my mammogram. Luck continued to be my partner, as my local Office Depot had stacks of "Komen" pink folders with the universally recognized pink ribbon embellished on the front. I bought every single one I could locate from all the area stores.

I made more than 150 folders with a one-page summary of the bill, compelling breast cancer facts, my tumor-hiding mammogram side by side with a mammogram showing how easy it is to spot a tumor in a fatty un-dense breast, and a drawing of a ruler displaying how big 4cm is. Just in case people didn't know it was the diameter of a golf ball. At the time I was very active in my local Komen for the Cure affiliate and was profoundly grateful when the Texas affiliates wrote a letter in support of the bill. It emphasized the importance of informing women about dense breast tissue. Both the Komen letter and a local magazine article about my story with pictures of my kids completed my handouts. I signed each cover letter "Thank You, Henda" with a fuchsia marker.

Leveraging the widespread association between breast cancer and pink, I decided that my marching uniforms for Austin would be dresses and jackets in all shades of pink. A quick stop at the local mall instantly expanded my wardrobe. It was show time! I was ready to show and share the story and picture of my right boob with every person I could get in front of—whether a parking attendant, aide, senator, representative, lobbyist, or assistant.

One-Legged at a Butt-Kicking Convention

A S YOU ARE BY now a specialist in breast density, let's kick up the curriculum. Get ready for the bull-dust class about Texas politics. One cannot make this stuff up! Hang with me for the next few pages because by the end, we can start a contract lobbyist firm specializing in fertilizer and elephant dung (a.k.a. total BS!).

The bill had two components. Part one informed and educated women about their breast density and the benefits of supplemental screening. Part two required insurance carriers to cover supplemental screening for women with dense breasts as part of their annual wellness exams. There was about a zero chance of passing the insurance part in a Republican-controlled house and senate with a conservative governor at the wheel. But the information and education part had a chance and was known as House Bill 834 (HB-834).

I also received a crash course on the timeline of passing bills and all the committees and hearings it had to successfully navigate in order to land on the governor's desk for signature. Thousands of bills die on the vine during each session, meaning they never make it to the governor before the 140 days of the regular legislative session runs out. In this case that crucial date was May 30, 2011.

In early March we filed a second bill in the house, HB-2102. It contained only the insurance portion to separate it from the more promising HB-834. Working two bills with their own timelines necessitated double the testifying and lobbying. I stuffed additional information inside my pink folders to clearly communicate the differences between the two and added a legend to keep all the numbers and nuances straight. When the session opened I thought I could dance quite well. Right. Let's take some more dance lessons! And while at it, let me learn to speak Texan real good, as I had no daylight to burn.

The best strategy was to defer to the professional lobbyists and seasoned political staff members, learning from them how to navigate the storm waters of Texas politics. I quickly discovered that the capitol cafeteria was a powerful place to linger with the intention of running into key people. My tactics paid off when some of the various allies I had made over repeated visits would text me to "show up" in the cafeteria whenever a critical aide or lobbyist had been spotted buying lunch. I had perfected my message and could flawlessly deliver the sound bites in less than two minutes. I rattled off my story over and over with no loss of enthusiasm all spring. It was draining, the reliving and retelling of those dark days after my cancer diagnosis to politicians' staff who were jaded by a system that had little room and even less time for a novice like me.

My fiercest supporter remained my *Midwest Academy* friend and mentor from the Texas Hold 'Em poker game. Douglas wasn't kidding when he assured me that I would need every special interest group to be either in favor of or at least not opposing the bills. Once again drawing on my background in sales and gut instinct, I tried to decipher which staff members for each representative and senator were the decision makers on what reached their boss's desk and got his or her attention. My friend made many introductory calls on my behalf, and without his guidance I would have had a very slim chance of succeeding. That said, he did withhold some essential information. He failed to tell me that the success of most bills also hinged on the elbow twisting, schmoozing, and lobbying during the off year between legislative sessions. A bill filed two weeks into the current session stood a less-than-zero chance of making it beyond filed status. He also didn't let me in on the secret of how "big money" rules Texas politics. With a state as large as Texas, running for office requires buckets of money like a federal campaign. Special interests are king, and I had no idea that Texas politics were in the same league as New York and California as far as complexity.

By the end of the 140 days of the 82nd Texas legislature on May 30, I would have earned the equivalent of a bachelor's degree in political science. The difference was that I earned it on the ground in combat instead of from books in a classroom. It was a war of attrition as I fought not with superior skill or strength, but instead with an unwavering faith in what was right. Not to mention clever resource management.

Since the first breast density law in the United States passed in Connecticut in 2009, a small army of seven women had evolved, all fighting on our individual state fronts. In addition to Texas, similar efforts by women like me were underway in Florida, Virginia, California, New York, and Missouri. We were all survivors of a laterstage diagnosis, our tumors were all undetected by mammograms, and we all had dense breast tissue. I felt incredible pressure to deliver the goods in a large, very red state. If Texas could pass a density bill, other states would leverage the momentum and the density snowball would get rolling.

For a bill to be signed by the governor and become law in Texas, it must pass with a majority vote in the house and senate. As both bills worked their way through the house, I would often get calls in Dallas at 7:00 a.m. from a staff member to come down to Austin to testify. Armed with my folders and always wearing a pretty pink dress, I would drop everything in Dallas for the three-hour drive to the capitol.

Testifying in front of the different house committees for more than a month was nerve-racking. I wrote out my testimony to maximize the six to eight minutes allocated to ensure that I didn't miss vital points. This was one time I was not depending on my ability to improvise, and I practiced my message until it evolved into a smooth delivery of why this legislation was necessary. Taking my place behind the podium in the different committee chambers, I was aware of a small red light blinking when I had neared my time. Each committee member had the chance to ask me follow-up questions. My outward calm belied my insides of twisted rubber bands ready to snap.

Before and after testifying I continued meandering the halls and handing out my pink folders to anybody in sight. Luck was often looking out for me. One time I walked in on the birthday party of a senior Democrat who also happened to be a breast cancer survivor. After telling her my story I could count on her vote! Good fortune was also on my team on another occasion when a veteran aide pulled me aside, tore off a piece of paper from her notebook, and wrote down about thirty names. She advised me to focus my efforts on them and their staff members, deeming them the real bigwigs at the capitol. I also had a short list of the main special interest lobbyists to target. The bill stood no chance without their support.

I was humbled by the large number of people I talked to who

were touched by cancer, whether personally or through their family and friends. Cancer was the common thread we shared, and it crossed all party lines and demographics.

Possum Pie for Dinner

I HAVE A FRIEND who says that a big sky opens our mind. Since transplanting myself to Texas the spectacular display of such a sky has rarely failed to render me speechless—whether a sunrise or sunset, the moon debuting, or white clouds dancing across its great expanse. After I left the capitol for Dallas I was often treated to an extraordinary sunset that made me feel like a VIP guest at the sun's farewell performance. It teased me with its reluctance to drop out of sight and rewarded me with several encores before taking a last bow. Hanging like a fireball in the west and streaking flares across the sky in Morse code, it brilliantly colored the wide-open spaces of nightfall in crimson.

I exhaled as I drove, letting go of more of the tension knotted in every corner of my being with each mile I clocked. My mind had permission to remove its shoes and wiggle itself loose from the confines I had stuck myself in to stay on message with all the players at the capitol. Nature's powerful presence on those nights was my private comfort guide. It assured me that the detours, twists, and turns were all part of it. As a train lover I recognized that it was never about the journey or the destination; it was choosing to board the train. I felt I was on a runaway express speeding down a steep mountain.

The soothing qualities of food always play a valuable part in my experiences, and the treks back and forth to Austin were no different. That spring and early summer I discovered roasted marrowbones from Durham, Wyoming, and the best fattoush salad this side of Lebanon. Even the Capitol Grill surprised me with fresh mozzarella and pesto on nutty bread. Left over from my radiation days, finding great Texas BBQ is still a prized pursuit, and I never miss an opportunity to unearth the next best brisket, ribs, and coleslaw.

Driving home from Austin, I almost always stopped at a barbecue joint near I-35 to sample their smoked meat and side dish specialties. I avoided the big chains and instead sought out the smaller mom & pop spots. Dressed in my pink ensemble and heels, I was used to being stared at as the drop-in alien. I once stopped near Abbott, Texas, (population 356), but it was not my lucky day because the slaw was out, the brisket cold, and the sauce neither smoky nor sweet. While enjoying some decent barbecue beans and ribs, I suddenly sensed that I was no longer

POSSUM PIE FOR DINNER

alone and felt two piercing eyes staring at me. After scanning the crowd my gaze shifted down to the ground beneath my dinner table and I came eye to eye with a sizable possum! I assumed that he had come for dinner as well, perhaps sensing how out of place we both were. As I didn't speak Possum, our silent conversation was a little limited, the exchange brief, and I never did get his recommendations for better brisket stops nearby. On my way out I mentioned to the server about the possum looking for scraps and was met with an effusive, "Hell, Honey! And you did not scream?" I just smiled, wanting to assure her that it takes politicians, not possums, to make me cry.

One Wheel Down and the Axle Dragging

THE BOEING 767 CABIN was dimly lit and silent as most of my fellow passengers were fast asleep. It was the summer of 2011, and my family and I were more than halfway into our six-hour flight from Anchorage back to Dallas after a vacation. We had spent the past two weeks in an RV touring the rugged land of the north. It was my second excursion to the wild and wonderful that defines Alaska in summer. I'd carried a fantasy about the quintessential American family vacation in an RV, as it didn't get any more white-picket fence than that in my mind! I rented the six-person deluxe model with a master bedroom, another queen bed above the driver's section, and living and dining room seats that collapsed into a double bed. Included were a small kitchen and bathroom. Snug would be a good word to describe it. Compact would also do it justice. Cramped out of my friggin' mind and trapped on wheels would be the honest picture.

When I ask my kids today what they remember most about the family vacation, they recall a similar picture. Apparently I appeared permanently pissed off the entire time. They tiptoed around the RV to not trip my crazy fuse, and generally felt that Mom was a bomb waiting to explode. We arrived in Alaska the first week in June, just days after the 82nd Texas legislature ran its course. I was burned out and mentally exhausted from my time impersonating a lobbyist and politician, especially the last hurried and stress-filled days of the session.

On May 25, five days before the clock ran out, I received a call to come to the capitol as soon as possible to testify in the senate. The senators on the state affairs committee were calling a special hearing immediately following the day's agenda to hear testimony in favor of Henda's Law. HB-834 (the education-only piece) had already died on the vine in the public health committee due to political agendas and special interests. To my surprise, HB-2102 (with the insurance component only) passed in the Texas house and was now on its way to the senate.

But there was a problem. The chances of passing Henda's Law in the senate were slim to none if this bill obligated insurance carriers to pay for the additional screening. In fact the governor threatened to veto the bill as it was. It left us no choice but to switch out the insurance provision with the information and education pieces from the defunct HB-834. Backroom politics, anyone?

We were running out of time to get anything signed at all. By then I felt like an NFL quarterback advancing the ball ten yards at a time with two minutes left in the game and a touchdown short of winning.

Compared to my house testimony, sitting around a very large table on the senate floor while being grilled by senators was up there with cleaning the outside windows of a skyscraper. It was completely terrifying, and great was my joy when it passed unanimously! However, the celebration was very short lived because the bill still had to go back to the house to be reconciled and revoted on the house floor as we had switched the verbiage.

By then it was May 29, with one day left to get Henda's Law signed by both the house and senate before time was up. The final tally of the house vote was Yes 136, No 5, Not Voting 2. As the last grains of sand fell through the top bubble of the hourglass, they sent the signed bill to the governor for his signature on May 30, 2011. It was the 140th day and just hours before it was too late. In hindsight I should have sought out a beach chair under a palm tree on a deserted island to regroup instead of ten days in an RV. I had to set up everyone's beds every night, break them down every morning, plot our route, prepare three meals a day, determine our grey water drops, do laundry for four people every other day, clean, and play tour guide and activities director. You probably would have been mad as hell too!

From our starting point in Anchorage we drove north to Talkeetna, a small Alaskan town in the shadow of Denali. Small, funky, and quaint, it was the launch pad for many adventurers wanting to conquer North America's tallest peak. Adding to my bracelets from everywhere, I picked up my oldest bracelet there. It dates back 50,000 years and I found it in a little shop in Talkeetna. It is solid silver with oval-shaped disks of wooly mammoth ivory tusks. As the tundra has been slowly melting, these tusks are coming to the surface. The locals use it to carve striking objects and jewelry. I fancy wearing this bracelet because it reminds me of the majesty of Alaska. When it encircles my wrist I feel tied to its land and spirit.

From there we carried on to Denali National Park and parked our mobile motel with views of the spectacular Alaska Range. It seemed almost sacrilegious to be in the presence of such grand views that few have the privilege to experience while filled with shadows and despair. Every day I awoke anxiously hoping that Governor Perry would sign the bill that day, and every night I went to sleep in anguish. I was a yo-yo being pulled back and forth, incapable of being present in God's country.

Growing up in South Africa close to nature gave me a tremendous appreciation for the untamed. Residing in the US, I had not found many truly unspoiled places like Alaska. Its grandeur and size overwhelmed me, and I could sense how nature only tolerated the human dwellings that dotted the landscape. It felt as if it stood ready at any time to engulf them. Being surrounded by eagles, bears, whales, and orcas reminded me of the necessity to have nature near me.

After Denali we headed south toward the Kenai Peninsula and my sour mood continued to fester. While watching the bald eagles in their effortless liftoffs and landings, I fantasized about feeding some of the people I'd met at the capitol in small bites to the eagles. I imagined them being airlifted to nests filled with little bald eagle hatchlings. I know—evil thoughts to be having while surrounded by glaciers, thick forests, and snowcapped mountain ranges.

Our next stop was Seward, another coastal community famous for the original mile zero of the Iditarod—The Last Great Race. I promptly added volunteering one day on the Iditarod to my bucket list. And I don't even like dogs! But the dogs running this race are fine athletes inspiring man to take on nature in an epic challenge. Together they cross 1,000 miles of the remotest, roughest, coldest terrain on the planet. Totally badass, if you ask me!

Orcas were joyously frolicking in the icy waters on our way to the Kenai Fjords National Park. While watching them I was having flashbacks of the strain of sitting in the gallery in the Texas house watching the final debate of HB-2102 before the vote. Our RV crisscrossed the great state of Alaska while I remained the dark storm cloud unable to snap out of my fear that I would fail. If the governor did not sign the bill, all the effort would be for nothing.

In Homer we fished for halibut in the ocean and for king salmon on a remote lake in the Alaskan wilderness that was only accessible by private seaplane. Our bush pilot was a rugged native and detoured to fly us over a glacier and across summer plains filled with moose, brown bears, and grizzly bears. We brought back to Dallas more than seventy pounds of halibut and salmon. After six months of "Henda's fish dishes," my kids suggested that we switch back to beef and chicken permanently! By the way, I'm not sure if you noticed the scene names in this section are dedicated to great Texan speak. I myself didn't know expressions like these and stole them off the internet.

At the end of our vacation we boarded our flight back to Dallas to head home on June 17. It was exactly two years from the day I had been lying in the OR waiting for a large chunk of cancer to be removed from my right breast. My phone rang at 4:00 p.m. as I handed my checked bags to the airline attendant. The bill had been signed into law! Certainly far from perfect, Texas women with dense breast tissue would now receive a letter, after having a mammogram, informing them of vital information that could potentially save their lives. Many Austin lobby chefs cooked up the final verbiage. If I wrote the legislation, I would have used simple English words and shorter sentences, and added a few Oxford commas.

2011 marked my conversion in becoming a pragmatist. I stopped condemning myself for not achieving complete perfection. If moving forward required a few steps back, I no longer gave myself ten lashings with a sjambok before bedtime. Giving it my best has become good enough. And then the chips must fall.

HB-2102 took effect on September 1, 2011, and was fully implemented in all mammogram facilities in Texas by January 1, 2012.

Henda's Law

If your mammogram demonstrates that you have dense breast tissue, which could hide abnormalities, and you have other risk factors for breast cancer that have been identified, you might benefit from supplemental screening tests that may be suggested by your ordering physician. Dense breast tissue, in and of itself, is a relatively common condition. Therefore, this information is not provided to cause undue concern, but rather to raise your awareness and to promote discussion with your physician regarding the presence of other risk factors, in addition to dense breast tissue. A report of your mammogram results will be sent to you and your physician. You should contact your physician if you have any questions or concerns regarding this report.

The Morning After

AND HERE I THOUGHT I was a hero! By early fall in 2011 I ran head-on into the Henda-haters. If only the law was simply identified as House Bill 2102. The backlash from the medical community was crushing. Didn't see it coming. I had planned on wearing a pink superhero cape for Halloween.

Radiologists embraced the disclosure, but many primary care physicians, internal medicine docs, and ob-gyns resented it. It forced changes to the status quo. Oh, and what do you know—also changes to the standard of care.

Many physicians didn't understand dense breast tissue either. Furthermore, they objected to the additional disclosure as it demanded more discussion time during a patient's wellness exam. Time that was not billable. And patients would need supplemental screening that might not be covered by the patients' insurance. I understood their pain and frustration and wanted to hire one of those little planes to fly around with a banner: The Governor Planned to Veto the Insurance!

But I had zero sympathy. Zippy zilch. They were not the ones dying. Some of us were. Watch me care about their discomfort. I knew that Henda's Law was imperfect. But I also completely believed that it would kick start meaningful conversations about how to screen for about half of all women with dense breasts.

My feelings were hurt by the backlash, but my skin was thick enough when I read the criticism on social media and the press. For a while I got a regular weekly fax notice from one ob-gyn advising me to stick to selling houses and stop trying to practice medicine. Week after week I slowly fed his message through my shredder. Friends and clients gladly shared their stories, good and bad, about asking their doctors about their breast density after they received the "You have dense breast tissue" letter.

As a breast cancer survivor I can vouch for how scary it is to be screened—before, during, and after. It is alarming to hear that you have dense breast tissue. Trust me. Being told you have a laterstage breast cancer is way scarier. *Girlfriends, you should embrace the knowledge and get to know the best way to care for those lovely boobies!* Regarding all cancers, I have never wavered in my belief that an early diagnosis is what we all deserve. That's where "survival" lives. I don't care who is scared and who is pissed off. My activism emerged from my anger about not having the opportunity to manage my breast care or an early cancer diagnosis. I'm still a little pissed off. And about that insurance veto—I was furious at the stupidity of politics for several years, as me and my gang in Austin tried in vain in 2013 and 2015 to get that portion of the bill passed.

Ta da! Which brings us to the 85th Texas legislature in 2017. Sweet revenge. I was not running the ball this time, and House Bill 1036 was in expert, professional lobbyist hands. But I was watching the play-by-play back in Dallas. The bill would cover 3D mammography during a woman's wellness exam. What the heck is 3D? Still far from peeing on a stick, it's the latest emerging technology in mammography. Does it catch all? No. Does it catch more tumors and penetrate dense breast tissue better? Yes. Do I sleep a little better at night? Yes. Am I a fan of Texas politics? Hell, no! In 2011 Texas was just the second state to pass breast density legislation. By the middle of 2017 only ten states in the United States were left without an enacted law, an introduced law, or active legislation of a bill regarding dense breast tissue. We surpassed the tipping point years before. The many grassroots efforts to change how we care for dense breasts are important, as it was (and is) about life and death. And we all choose life. Boobs and all. Who matters most to me? The women who call and email me to share their stories about their breast cancer, annual screenings, dense breasts, and lumps. And the ones who ask me to help them. Their faith in my guidance through this convoluted nightmare has become my most cherished way of connection. Its power brings me comfort and validates that together we are strong and will survive. I also care about the many hundreds of thousands who think I'm just some breast law without a face and story.

www.ingramcontent.com/pod-product-compliance
Lightning Source LLC
Chambersburg PA
CBHW060513280326
41933CB00014B/2948